I0470964

Nursing Career Development

Career Development Tools for Nurses and Hospitals

LOUISE D. JAKUBIK

Louise D. Jakubik, PhD, RN-BC
President and Chief Learning Officer
Nurse Builders
Philadelphia, PA

First Edition

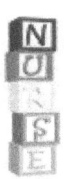

Nurse Builders, Philadelphia, PA

Published by:
Nurse Builders
7715 Crittenden Street, Box 350
Philadelphia, PA 19118
www.nursebuilders.net

All rights reserved. No part of this book may be reproduced or transmitted in any form or by any means, electronic or mechanical, including photocopying, recording or by any information storage or retrieval system without written permission from the author, except for inclusion of brief quotations in a review.

Copyright © 2014 by Louise D. Jakubik.
First edition.
Printed in the United States of America.

Dedication

For those readers who are beginning your careers as a professional nurse, welcome to this remarkable profession. I look forward to helping you to navigate your career journey! For those readers who are seasoned nursing professionals, I hope that this book has a role in re-energizing your career journey. For those who approach this read as a way to learn more about developing nurses within the context of the organizational workforce, thank you for listening and for working to develop this most precious resource: our nursing professionals.

This book is dedicated to nurses and to nursing. Thank you for what you do. You are my heroes. You are the reason I do what I do every day to support you and promote you in your practice and professional development. And thank you to the profession of nursing for being a vocation and a career that has both excited and humbled me from the start. It is through service to patients, families, and nurses that

4 | *Nursing Career Development*

I have had the good fortune to develop my own career in nursing and to help others to do the same. I am in awe of this profession we call nursing and can't imagine doing anything else!

About the Author

Dr. Louise Jakubik, PhD, RN-BC is a nursing career development expert. She is passionate about developing nurses in their careers and helping the organizations in which they work to embed systems, structures, and values that promote nursing career development. She is the President and Chief Learning Officer of Nurse Builders, a nursing education firm that specializes in developing nurses and nursing organizations through continuing education, certification review, onboarding consultation, curriculum design, and both practice and research consultation. Dr. Jakubik received her BSN and MSN in acute and chronic nursing of children from University of Pennsylvania, and her PhD in nursing from Widener University. Her research agenda focuses on mentoring practices and benefits for nurses and the organizations in which they work. Dr. Jakubik has held roles in nursing including staff nurse, pediatric nurse practitioner, clinical nurse specialist and nurse entrepreneur. She is a frequent speaker on a variety of leadership and clinical topics including pediatric nursing certification review, test taking, pediatric laboratory interpretation, mentoring, career development, and innovation in nursing education.

CONTENTS

8 | *Nursing Career Development*

Introduction

I've often wished that the first day of a nurse's career started with receiving a *career toolbox* to assist in navigating his or her professional life as a nurse. This book is designed to do just that. Whether you are a novice or a seasoned nurse, this book will provide you with valuable information about how specific *career development tools* in your *career toolbox* can unlock keys to success in your personal career journey. More importantly, though, this book will outline how these *career development tools* are essential for not only individual nurses, but also for hospitals to use in partnership with their nurses to develop careers in nursing.

This book will explore specific *career development tools* for developing a career in nursing from start to finish. This book is divided into ten chapters, each exploring a specific *career development tool* for career development. Each *career development tool* chapter contains two sections: part I for the individual nurse and part II for hospitals.

Part I explores the role of the individual nurse in using a specific *career development tool* to develop his or her career in nursing. Part II explores the role of the hospital in using each *career development tool* to develop its nurses throughout their careers.

These *career development tools* are not secrets. They are not things you've never heard of or considered. *Career development tools* are catalysts of career development which are generally underutilized by both individual nurses and the organizations in which they work. Furthermore, their strategic power is generally underestimated in their ability to enhance and promote the career of a professional nurse. In this book, we'll explore what exactly these *career development tools* are and how to use them so that individual nurses and hospitals can unleash the power of these career development catalysts.

At the end of each chapter, you'll have the opportunity to complete a *career development exercise* where you can explore how you as an individual nurse can use the *career development tool* in your own professional life. If you are in a position to lead a hospital career development initiative, there is also a *career development exercise* at the end of each chapter for you to consider how your hospital could play a more strategic role in the career development of individual nurses using the specific *career development tool* in that chapter.

How to Use this Book

Whether you are a student nurse, a novice nurse just entering practice, or a seasoned nurse, this book is for you. Think about who your *nursing idols* are. Who do you look up to and want to be like? Have you ever wondered how he or she got to their position or role? Is your *nursing idol*:

- an expert clinical nurse or an expert charge nurse on your unit
- an advanced practice nurse at your hospital whose patient assessment and management skills are excellent
- a faculty member who taught you during your formative years as a student nurse
- a nurse manager or executive whose leadership style you aspire to emulate
- a nurse author or speaker who inspires you

Whoever your *nursing idol* happens to be, I promise you that he or she used many of the *career development tools* outlined in this book to develop in nursing. This book is designed to expose you to the menu of nursing career development strategies, called *career development tools*, which are available for you to use throughout your career as you develop as a professional nurse. Use the *career development exercises* at the end of each chapter to consider how you might begin to employ the specific *career development tool* discussed in the chapter. Many of these *career development tools* are free and readily available to you. All you have to do is start to use them.

If you are a nursing professional development expert or nurse administrator who is working to develop nurses within your organization, this book will provide you with an overview of specific ways you and your hospital can facilitate nurses' access to the *career development tools* they need to develop throughout their careers in nursing. Nurses and their employers both benefit from nurses being developed to their full potential and having the *career development tools* to accomplish just that.

Think of this book as a road map for a career in nursing. It provides the map for how to develop yourself and others as professional nurses.

Warning -- Disclaimer

This book is designed to provide you with the information you need to either develop yourself or others as professional nurses. Every effort has been made to make this book as accurate as possible. The information contained in this book is designed to be representative of contemporary literature and the author's expertise in developing and mentoring thousands of nurses across the United States for success in nursing.

16 | Nursing Career Development

Chapter 1
Making a Commitment

Part 1: Nurses

Developing your career in nursing really is up to you. Career building by definition requires that you seek out paths to advancement by acquiring additional knowledge and skills. Additionally, attaining additional roles (e.g. preceptor, charge nurse, committee chair), responsibilities (e.g. teaching, chart audits), and positions (e.g. nurse manager, nurse educator) are also key ways to position yourself to advance your career in nursing.

Career versus job?

One of the challenges for nurses as they consider developing their careers in nursing is, in fact, how they view being a nurse. Is being a nurse a job or a career? The answer to that question really is a state of mind. It's a question that needs to be asked and answered at different points in time throughout our careers in nursing. And at different points in one's life as a professional nurse, the answer may vary. And that's okay. In fact, that really is one of the best things about nursing: that you can change shifts, work hours, roles, and even specialties throughout your working years to meet personal and professional needs and goals at a given point in time. When you are pursuing your graduate degree and have young children, that part-time weekend position may truly be "just a job" while you are pursuing your life and career goals. At other times, you will experience the excitement of feeling your vocation as you are meeting a patient's need, answering a student's question, or addressing a clinical or research question. The flexibility that nursing provides to be able to navigate our professional and personal lives is truly unique.

So what differentiates a job from a career? A job is generally task or trade oriented with monetary compensation as a reward. A career involves personal and professional enhancement, monetary compensation, and some measure of intrinsic reward. Careers can also be vocations.

What is Your Slice of Nursing?

Developing your career in nursing requires time and energy. But it does not have to be overwhelming either. In my opinion a key ingredient in developing your career in nursing is to figure out what it is about nursing that excites you. What are you passionate about? Pay attention to that. That is your *slice of nursing*. Look for how that *slice of nursing* that can be cultivated in you. For me, I recognized early on that I really loved clinical practice but at the same time I was drawn to the academic aspects of nursing. I liked writing, teaching, and questioning practice. So I looked to expose myself to experiences that were practice-focused and included some of the academic components I really enjoyed. When leaders tried to pull me away from the bedside, I knew that wasn't the role for me because the clinical care was what really excited me about nursing. Today, while I no longer clinically take care of patients, nurses whom I teach all across the country will tell you how focused on clinical practice I am, and how dedicated I am to serving nurses who take care of patients at the bedside. It's what I am passionate about. It's my *slice of nursing*.

Once you determine your *slice of nursing* you will be able to focus your career development efforts on those knowledge, skills, and roles in that *slice of nursing* that may be ones you can cultivate today or years from today. No matter what, it is a focus area where you can start your career development journey.

Career Development Exercise

1. How do you see your position in nursing at the present time? Is it a career or a job?

_____

_____

2. What is your *slice if nursing*? Remember this is the piece of nursing that ignites your passion and excitement. List the aspects that you enjoy:

_____

_____

_____

_____

3. Are you ready to begin to build your career in nursing?

_____

Part 2: Hospitals

Do you have the right philosophy?

Hospitals, by their very nature have a culture and a set of values that drive their actions. These values and organizational culture determine where human and financial resources are allocated and are reinforced by the leaders through role modeling. So the first question for you to ask yourself as an organizational leader is whether or not your hospital values developing nurses? And if it does not, why not? Is your hospital one that worries if it develops nurses, that they will leave leading to increased nursing vacancies? Is your hospital committed to developing nurses but does not perceive it has the resources; either human or financial, to do so? Generally, the answers to these questions are varied and deeply embedded in organizational history and culture. But remember, each leader has a role is setting the organizational tone, culture, and values through role modeling and through his or her own actions. So the fact that you are reading this book as a leader in clinical practice, staff education, and/or management means that you will be equipped with the tools that you need to begin to develop nurses in their careers in nursing.

Are you willing to make the investment?

A common misperception among organizational leadership is that it's labor and cost intensive to develop nurses. And while it can be, it does not have to be so. In this section, I will ask those of you who are organizational leaders to dig deep and ask yourself if you and your hospital want to create a culture that develops nurses. Do you want to be known for helping nurses to cultivate their knowledge, skills, and careers? Are you as a leader and as an organization comfortable with the consequences that nurses might develop and exit the hospital for other opportunities, while others will be attracted to your hospital because it will be known for developing and growing its nurses?

I would argue that hospitals and organizational leaders are called to develop their nurses. These nurses are the seeds that each hospital is entrusted with. As the gardener, the hospital and its leaders are entrusted the role of cultivating the organizational soil and climate that will create the garden in which these nurse seedlings can be nourished, grow and eventually bloom.

I learned as a young clinical leader in nursing that nurses are attracted to people and places that develop them. As a young nurse leader, I always tried to start any conversation that involved constructive feedback with these words: "My role and my intention is to build and develop you as a nurse. I have no stake in tearing you down." I also lived those words. I modeled them at every opportunity. I still do. You see, developing people is a powerful attractor. Most of us want to be developed and to grow and we want to be around people who will grow us up rather than tearing us down. Nurse leaders (e.g. clinical nurses, nurse educators, nurse executives, etc.) who grow and develop those whom they serve, attract nurses to them and are magnets for talent.

The hospital and its leaders have the power by setting the tone, the culture, the values, and the role modeling to set the stage as an organization that grows and develops nurses. If you want this type of environment for your nurses, this book will help you to fill your *career development toolbox* with strategies to just that.

Career Development Exercise

1. Do you perceive that your organization values developing nurses? If so, how is that demonstrated? If not, how is that demonstrated?

_____

_____

_____

_____

2. Are you as a leader ready to develop other nurses through your actions and the systems and structures you and others can put in place? And if so, what skills and resources do you bring to this role?

_____

_____

_____

_____

_____

_____

_____

Chapter 2
Learning and Growing: Continuing Education and Formal Academic Education

Background

Continuing education (CE) and professional development can be categorized into two main areas: (1.) continuing education programs and (2.) formal academic education programs. State boards of nursing establish both the academic minimum requirements and continuing education requirements for initial licensure and license renewal. These requirements vary from state to state.

Part 1: Nurses

Continuing Education

Continuing education (CE) is an important avenue to develop knowledge and skills throughout one's career as a nurse. Ideally, CE is targeted to a nurse's experience and knowledge level.

0-2 Years of Experience:

Novice and advanced beginner nurses in the first one to two years of practice should be able to meet their learning needs through unit-based and/or hospital-based CE. Nurses at this level are gathering beginning content knowledge about nursing practice and, therefore, the more basic content offered at the unit level and generic content offered at the hospital-level are ideal for this level of nursing knowledge and skill development.

Two Years and Beyond:

Nurses with 2 or more years of experience generally benefit more from regional and national specialty-based CE. Typically, these types of CE are run by either professional nursing organizations or conference management companies. Generally, nurses at this level require more in-depth, specialty-based knowledge and skills provided by nursing content experts at these regional and national conferences. These types of forums provide not only more advanced knowledge and skill enrichment, but also career and role enhancement through the networking opportunities that these types of CE forums include. Conferences that are run by professional nursing organizations frequently provide opportunities for nurses to join committees, task forces, or run for elected office in the professional organization at the local or national level. Both types of regional and national specialty-based continuing education conferences typically provide opportunities to present poster and oral presentations, which are also great forums for networking.

Additionally, there are a variety of self-learning options for nurses seeking additional specialty education which include web-based self-learning modules, journal CE articles, and audio and video CE. These options allow nurses to self-direct and self-pace their learning while obtaining more in-depth, specialty-based nursing CE. There is generally wide variability as to the quality of these options and, therefore, nurses and hospitals must discern the quality of a particular self-learning product. This can be done by considering the author's level of expertise (e.g. credentials and experience in the content area); publisher's reputation; overall quality of the content (e.g. typographical errors, appearance); and currency of the information (e.g. references within the past 5 years).

Formal Academic Education Programs

Traditional formal academic education degrees for nurses include bachelor's, master's, and doctoral degrees. Obtaining additional degrees in nursing prepares nurses for promotion and additional role attainment in nursing.

Making the Decision

Many nurses really struggle with whether or not to obtain an advanced degree and, if so, which one to obtain. In some cases, nurses are required to obtain an advanced degree due to employer requirements. For instance some Magnet hospitals and Magnetjourneying hospitals are requiring nurses whose highest level of preparation is a diploma or associate's degree in nursing, to achieve a bachelor's degree in nursing within a given time frame in order to remain employed at the organization. Other state and national nursing accreditation requirements have required nurses in existing roles in advanced practice nursing (e.g. clinical nurse specialist) to achieve additional certification and/or academic preparation at the advanced practice level. Some nurses know they want to advance their education and their role in nursing and seek out additional education toward that end. Whatever the reason nurses seek out advanced education, there are several issues to consider prior to making the leap.

Which Degree? Which Academic Institution?

The central question to answer prior to choosing a particular degree and academic institution is: What do you want to do or to be? In other words: What is your professional goal as an outcome of obtaining this degree?

Hospital Required Degree

If your goal is to meet a hospital requirement for obtaining a degree such as a bachelor's degree, then your basic considerations are surrounding choosing a program that is convenient, and of reasonable cost and quality. So those are the factors that you would consider when choosing a particular program. You also want to look at factors like graduation rate and time frame. If for instance, you are required to get a bachelor's degree by a given date then you want to be sure that the academic institution has a reputation of moving its students through the program within your identified time frame.

Role Attainment

If your goal is to obtain a particular role in the future (e.g. nurse manager, nurse executive, nurse educator) then you need to consider what the requirements are for that role within your organization, your state, and the nation as a whole. You may find that the requirements vary. For instance in some hospitals, it is commonplace for nurse managers to be required to have a master's degree, while in others a bachelor's degree may be the minimum requirement. In some hospitals, nurse educators are required to hold master's degrees and/or certificates specifically in nursing education. Other hospitals require a master's degree only in no particular specialization. And other hospitals do not require an advanced degree, but rather require interest and experience in nursing education.

Advanced Practice Preparation

If your goal is to become prepared to work in the future as an advanced practice nurse (APN), it is important that you explore those roles. It's a good idea to talk with practicing APNs to learn more about their roles. Perhaps you can set up a day to shadow an APN to see what the role is really like. APN roles vary greatly. And it is important to try to match your goals and desires to the type of APN role you pursue.

Nurse practitioners are primarily patient care providers. They typically perform history and physical examinations and write orders with a collaborating physician. They may work in a primary care or specialty outpatient practice setting where they are required to do some evening and weekend shifts. They may work in the hospital setting on a team where they work a more traditional work day without weekends or evening requirements. Many neonatal intensive care APNs work 24-hour shifts with days off in between. And many surgical APNs start their surgical day in the hospital at 6am.

Clinical nurse specialists more commonly focus on aspects of nursing role components like: change agency, research, quality improvement, and education (patient, family, and/or nurses). Typically, clinical nurse specialists work a traditional work week with business hours.

Nurse anesthetists generally work on an anesthesia team taking patient histories, managing patient's airways, and administering medications in either a procedural area or an operating room. Nurse anesthetists work when surgical suites are open which generally starts as early as 7am or earlier. The number of days per week and hours per day that a nurse anesthetist works may vary from practice to practice.

All of these factors from the type of work to the setting for practice, to the hours and flexibility are important factors for you to consider ahead of time as you are considering making the decision to go back to school to advance your career in nursing. It is important to consider what the roles require in terms of your professional work and your personal life.

Career Development Exercise

1. How many years of experience do you have in your specialty?

_____

2. Using the guidelines in this chapter (see pages 32-33), what type of conferences should you target to attend?

_____

_____

3. Take some time in the next hours or days to search for continuing education (CE) that will meet your needs. List them below.

_____

_____

_____

_____

4. Would you consider attending one or more of the CEs listed above in #3? What's your time frame to accomplish that?

_____

_____

_____

Part 2: Hospitals

Continuing Education

Continuing education (CE) is a hot topic in hospitals. Issues range from cost to infrastructure to human resources and beyond. Nursing educators and managers in hospitals can perform a baseline needs assessment by identifying: (1.) existing CE content (both internally and externally); (2.) nurses' knowledge and skills needs; and (3.) gaps between existing content and learning needs. Once this assessment is conducted, nursing leadership should identify ways to fill the gaps with new programming (either internal or external). Then, the curriculum content for CE is established.

The next step is to create a framework or methodology for how nurses will be moved through the CE curriculum content in a planned and organized way. Consideration should include matching the nurses' experience level to the types of CE as described on pages 32-33. Once this framework is established it should be shared throughout the organization so that everyone is aware of the approach to meeting nurses' learning needs through the curriculum content.

The key to success in CE for hospitals is that the content is built around knowledge and skills needs and that nurses are deliberately moved through the curriculum at the appropriate time with regard to their experience level. Such an approach facilitates the nurse growing and developing throughout a career in nursing rather than feeling like knowledge and skill development is haphazard or otherwise deficient.

Nursing leaders in education, practice, and management must assure that they are continually arming themselves with information obtained through CE and participation at the local and national professional organizations in their practice area. As leaders, they must also set the example for the importance of staying up to date and for benchmarking and networking with others in their specialty areas.

Formal Academic Education Programs

A more educated nursing workforce will naturally enhance the quality of the organization and promote succession planning. Hospitals have a role in promoting nurses going back to school to advance their education for its own sake. Hospitals also must identify young stars in nursing and encourage them to advance their education in order to be ready for future role advancement.

Tuition reimbursement is one way that hospitals can support nurses in advancing in their academic education. It is also an excellent recruitment and retention strategy. Tuition reimbursement programs often require a minimum number of months (typically 6-12) of employment prior to eligibility and may also have a requirement for ongoing employment after the reimbursement period or degree completion. Tuition reimbursement is a *career development tool* that not only helps organizations to recruit and retain nurses, but also promotes nurses' satisfaction, all while building a more educated and more invested workforce.

Many hospitals are partnering with academic institutions to offer onsite, local, and/or distance-learning academic degree completion programs, particularly at the baccalaureate level. These are partnership opportunities that create a win-win for the hospital and the university because they provide ongoing classes of students for the university while assisting the hospital to meet its organizational goals of advancing towards a baccalaureate prepared nursing workforce. These types of partnerships have been modeled across the country and will certainly continue to grow.

One important way that hospitals can build a culture of advancing nurses in higher education is for its leaders to role model it. If leadership in nursing does not attain advanced education in nursing, then it's difficult for the organization to maintain that advanced education in nursing is a value for the organization. Organizations that wish to promote baccalaureate, master, and doctoral degree completion in nursing must require that their nursing leaders attain those degrees as well. It is amazing to me how contagious advanced education can be. One or two key leaders can set the bar and create the impetus for others in the leadership group to go back and further their education.

I obtained my master's degree at 24 years old and my doctoral degree at 34 years old. (And yes I had a life. Though I am not always sure how I fit it all in. I got married at 23 and gave birth to my two children at 29 and 31, all while working full time and going to school after my first child was born. Today the kids are 9 and 11 years and my husband and I have been married for 17 years.) At the time when I got my master's degree I remember feeling like it was not a common thing to do and that I was the youngest person getting a master's degree by a good bit. I remember leaders in nursing who actually discouraged me. (I realize now that they were probably threatened by me as a young person pursuing an advanced degree.)

Fast forward 7 years when I was starting my doctoral degree at 30 years of age, there were young nurses and middle-aged nurses all around me who had gone back to school and started and many finished their master's degrees. By the time I started my doctoral degree it was a cultural norm to get a master's degree. The world of nursing, at least my local part of it, had changed and changed for the better.

Starting my doctoral degree at 30, I was cautiously optimistic. I had an infant daughter at the time and figured I'd give it a shot and see how I could juggle working full time, being a mom and wife and starting a doctoral program. It was actually fun! It gave me a new challenge and one evening a week out of the house and out of the office early to work on my own professional goals.

Again, at the time I had few nursing examples in my world with doctoral degrees and I felt like few supported me or even knew what I was doing or why I was doing it. (I knew that I had maxed out my knowledge and skills in some areas as a nursing leader. I felt that the doctoral education would prepare me to be a better resource to the nurses I served.)

Fast forward to today, ten years later, and nurses are pursuing doctorates at all age and experience levels. And what's most exciting is that I know hosts of nurses who are either contemplating the start of a doctoral program, actually applying for a doctoral program, or actively pursuing their doctoral education!

The point is that our nursing culture changes. And sometimes we are each part of the change. So taking the leap to achieve your bachelor's or master's or doctoral degree may start the momentum not only for you, but also for those around you who decide to join you on the journey. I truly believe that nursing leaders have a responsibility to set the standard by advancing themselves professionally through formal education in nursing.

Career Development Exercise

1. Perform a baseline education needs assessment. Consider the following:

    a. Summarize your existing CE content (both internally and externally):

_____

_____

    b. Summarize your nurses' knowledge and skills needs:

_____

_____

    c. Summarize the gaps between existing CE content and learning needs:

_____

_____

2. Does your hospital offer tuition reimbursement? If so, what is the policy?

_____

_____

3. How does or how can your hospital use formal education as a job satisfier?

_____

_____

Chapter 3
Getting Certified

Part 1: Nurses

Becoming certified in a nursing subspecialty is a professional accomplishment. It's a nationally valid and reliable measure of an individual nurse's command of the content area to support specialty nursing practice. It denotes a level of nursing content knowledge that brands you as a practicing specialty nurse. Nursing certifications exist at the generalist level (diploma, associate's degree, and baccalaureate) and advanced level (advanced practice). Some roles in nursing require certification either governed by the state board of nursing or by a particular employer.

No matter whether certification is required or optional, there is no question that nursing specialty certification elevates the level of nursing practice for individual nurses and the organizations in which the work. Hospitals who have been designated as 'Magnet hospitals' by the American Nurses Credentialing Center's (ANCC) Magnet

Recognition Program, have a documented higher rate of certified nurses than non-Magnet hospitals. These Magnet hospitals are among the best hospitals in the country. And the higher rate of certified nurses is believed to be one component of these hospitals' success.

So what are the benefits of becoming certified in my nursing subspecialty?

The individual benefits to getting certified in your nursing subspecialty are numerous. The most important reason to become certified is for your own personal gratification at knowing that you have achieved the mark of excellence that certification denotes. Additionally, being certified provides you with an avenue for professional advancement. Many employers will look at certification as an asset that puts you above other candidates for positions such as clinical instructor, committee chair, and unit educator. Nursing certification is often a pathway to further professional and academic advancement. Many nurses tell me they are ready for the next professional challenge after studying, preparing for and achieving their nursing subspecialty certification. Some go onto get an additional certificate or certification in nursing. Others go on to enroll in a nursing bachelor's or master's degree program.

So how do I know when to get certified?

The decision about when to seek national nursing subspecialty certification is largely an individual decision with regard to personal readiness. However, one place to start is to go to the exam website and review the minimum requirements for practice, experience, and educational preparation. Most of the national subspecialty certifications at the generalist level will require a minimum of one to two years of nursing practice experience in the subspecialty. At the advanced practice level, many certification exams are required for entry into practice and, therefore, the requirements are focused more on completion of the required master's degree at an accredited college or university in the specialty area. Once you've reviewed the minimum requirements for nursing subspecialty certification, it is time to decide on a timeline to prepare for and schedule your exam. There are many resources available to help you prepare which include: live and self-paced review courses, text books, practice questions books, study cards, and study groups.

How do I decide which nursing specialty certification to pursue?

As a general rule, it makes the most sense to first pursue the nursing specialty certification that is most closely tied to your practice area. So for instance, pediatric nurses should pursue certification as a pediatric nurse and medical-surgical nurses should pursue certification as a medical-surgical nurse. At times, nurses working in highly specialized areas like pediatric critical care, decide to purse certification as a pediatric nurse first prior to certification as a pediatric critical care nurse. Nurses who choose this route often tell me that they gain confidence by first studying for the more general exam related to their specialty before studying for the often more challenging exam related to their critical care subspecialty.

It is important to remember that as you branch out in your career, you may add additional specialties to your practice. For instance, a medical-surgical nurse who is promoted into a nurse manager role joins the specialty of nursing administration. It is, therefore, necessary at some point to consider certification in nursing administration to support the knowledge base in this particular role component. So as a nurse adds role components beyond his or her own core practice area, he or she should consider obtaining the additional certifications for those specialty areas. Having those certifications helps to demonstrate a nurse's specialty knowledge and is an achievement within that nursing specialty.

Career Development Exercise

1. List your nursing subspecialties below:

_____

_____

2. List your certifications below:

_____

_____

3. List the benefits for you to pursue additional certification:

_____

_____

4. What nursing subspecialty certification could you pursue? What is your timeline?

_____

_____

_____

5. What steps will you take in the next month to pursue becoming certified?

_____

_____

_____

_____

Part 2: Hospitals

There is no doubt that certification is a hot topic in the nursing profession and among hospitals in general. Hospital administrations understand the value of certification to national recognition programs and accreditation. The challenge for nursing leadership in hospitals is to create a culture that fosters certification in an ongoing way.

A culture of certification starts with the institutional supports a hospital puts in place such as incentives, rewards, and recognition that are an essential element of supporting and maintain such a culture. These types of supports include providing paid time to attend a review course, providing financial support for review course and exam fees, and may even include bonuses or promotions based on holding and maintaining nursing specialty certification. Low cost ways to promote certification include holding a certification fair during *Nurses' Week* where information about certification is available for various specialties. Most certification exam publishers will send free pamphlets or other materials to promote their certification exams. Furthermore, posters or handouts can be made to outline the hospital's tuition reimbursement and/or certification reward policies.

Obviously organizational resources are finite, but a hospital that holds nursing specialty certification as a high priority is one that puts supports in place for nurses to achieve and maintain their nursing specialty certification. We as individuals and as organizations demonstrate our values through our actions.

Organizational leaders must be role models for nursing specialty certification. Leaders have an obligation to demonstrate the value of certification through their own certification credentials.

Organizational leaders can do a lot to promote a culture of nursing certification by celebrating certification and certified nurses.

Recognition is a powerful thing. Some people don't like it, but most do. And recognition is something that does not really cost much, yet has tremendous value to the person who is being recognized. Examples of nursing certification recognition and celebration could include an annual certification breakfast or lunch to honor certified nurses throughout the hospital or a periodic awards ceremony to recognize newly certified nurses. Such celebrations are not necessarily expensive, yet the value added to the organization and the individual nurses can be immeasurable. Becoming certified is invigorating. And the momentum and energy created from a group of nurses becoming certified in tandem is simply amazing. Hospitals should celebrate this and hold it up as an example of excellence in nursing practice.

Career Development Exercise

1. How do you and other organizational leaders support certification in terms of actions/values?

_____

_____

2. List at least 2 ways you and your colleagues as organizational leaders could better support certification:

_____

_____

3. How does your hospital structurally support certification in terms of policies and procedures for certification?

_____

_____

_____

4. List at least 2 ways that your hospital could structurally support certification in terms of new or existing policies and procedures:

_____

_____

_____

_____

Chapter 4
Mentor and Be
Mentored

Part 1: Nurses

M*entoring* is a gift.   It is gift that we should each hope to receive throughout our careers and one that I truly believe each of us is called to give repeatedly and often throughout our careers. *Mentoring* is one of the most powerful *career development tools* that any nurse can experience.   It is no wonder that the rates of mentoring experiences are high among nurse leaders (Vance & Olson, 1998).

Mentoring in nursing is a career developmental relationship among an experienced nurse, a less experienced nurse, and the organization in which they work. It is intentional, long-term and involves an experience differential.   *Mentoring* in nursing involves specific mentoring practices (facilitated by the mentor) which are associated with six mentoring benefits for the protégé (Jakubik, 2007, 2008, Jakubik, Eliades, Gavriloff, & Weese, 2011). *Mentoring practices* are specific career developmental phenomena that are facilitated by the individual mentor. (Weese, Jakubik, Huth, & Eliades, in press). *Mentoring benefits* are those positive outcomes of the mentoring relationship that are experienced by the protégé, the mentor, and/or the organization (Zey, 1993).

It is your responsibility to be a mentor to other nurses. Research demonstrates that mentoring begets mentoring; that those who are mentored will become mentors (Jakubik, 2008, Jakubik, Eliades, Gavriloff, & Weese, 2011; Weese, Jakubik, Huth, & Eliades, 2013 in press). So by doing your part by being a mentor to other nurses, you are potentially increasing the number of mentors for future nurses.

Where do I begin to become a mentor?

Characteristics of good mentors include: role model, knowledgeable, skilled, patient, other-focused, respected, and trustworthy. Essentially, good mentors possess characteristics that others want to emulate. So by striving for excellence in your current nursing role, you will have many of the characteristics that a nurse mentor needs.

You can mentor other nurses informally or through a formal mentoring program provided by your hospital or through professional organizations that sponsor mentoring programs. A good place to start out as a new mentor is to examine what nursing knowledge and skills you are really good at and really enjoy sharing. Typically, mentors excel when they are sharing role components at which they excel. Of course, many of us have benefited from a nurse mentor who represented the total package of what we wanted to become as a nurse one day. Those generalist mentors are ones that we benefit from when we are starting in a new role.

Seeking Out a Mentor

It should be your aim to seek out being mentored throughout your career. Typically, nurses need different mentors for different career developmental needs throughout a career in nursing. At the start of a new role (e.g. staff nurse, nurse educator, nurse manager) we generally need a mentor who emulates the entire package of what that role embodies. As we grow in our careers, we typically need different mentors for different skill development. For instance, one mentor might be a "research mentor" who shows us how to read and analyze a research article and later includes us as part of a research investigation team. Another mentor might be our "education mentor" who guides us through presenting our first unit-based education presentation.

So how do I find a mentor?

Nurse mentors have a tendency to seek out protégés to mentor. However, nurse mentors are also often very busy so it's important to position yourself as an excellent choice as a future protégé. Characteristics of good protégés include: hard-worker, demonstrate follow-through, trustworthy, responsive, and accepts constructive feedback. Research shows that the benefits of mentoring are not related to whether the mentoring relationship is formal or informal, but rather the quality of the relationship is what is most important (Jakubik, 2008; Jakubik et al, 2011). So don't be concerned about whether you find a mentor through a formal mentoring program or not. Personally, I have found mentoring to be an organic process. I have collected protégés and mentors informally as the mutual benefits have presented themselves and as the personalities seemed to click.

Career Development Exercise

1. List the names of the nurses you are currently mentoring and specifically what you are doing:

_____

_____

_____

2. List at least one nurse who you could seek out to mentor whom you know would benefit:

_____

3. How might you start the mentoring relationship with the nurse you've identified?

_____

_____

_____

4. What needs do you have that could be fulfilled by a nurse mentor?

_____

_____

_____

5. Name a nurse or nurses who could be a mentor for you to assist you in developing your career:

_____

_____

_____

6. What steps will you take to make a mentor connection with the nurse(s) you've identified to mentor you?

_____

_____

_____

Part 2: Hospitals

Creating a mentoring culture for nurses is the responsibility of organizations and organizational leaders. A mentoring culture is one in which mentoring and developing people is an organizational value that is evidenced in the way leaders develop their people and in the ways in which the organization invests human and financial resources in developing people. Mentoring cultures hold those accountable who diminish others.

The value of a mentoring culture to a hospital is limitless. Mentoring cultures prevent peer bullying because in mentoring cultures, bullying is counter-cultural. Cultures that promote and foster mentoring naturally repel bullying behaviors. Mentoring cultures promote professional development and succession planning in nursing (Jakubik, 2008; Jakubik et al, 2011). Hospitals owe it to their human resources to create an environment in which they can flourish. It benefits not only the individuals, but also the organization by fostering people with the very best knowledge and skills for the workforce.

Creating a culture of mentoring can take many forms including: adoption of mentoring as a value-set by senior organizational executives, executive and middle management development, institutional mentoring systems and structures, adopting formal mentoring programs, and promoting informal mentoring. Organizations may use a variety of these strategies and may implement them in different ways.

A key ingredient in building an organization's mentoring culture is for the organization's leadership to adopt a values system that includes mentoring. Organizational values are held, modeled, and communicated through words and actions by senior executives. So in order to create a mentoring culture for an organization, it is essential that this value is adopted at the very top of the organization. However, mentoring cultures can be built at the local level by those in middle management. The key in mentoring cultures is that the leadership demonstrates in words, actions, systems and structures that mentoring is the expectation and the value. Managers, leaders and workers who hold this value will naturally hold accountable those whose actions undermine or fail to promote mentoring.

Leaders have a large role in creating the culture. So embedding the value of mentoring in executive and middle managers is essential. Developing executive and middle managers in their own skills and communicating the organizational value of mentoring is critical. Management has an essential role in communicating in words and actions what the organizational values are and in setting the stage for expectations of leadership and staff at the local level. Providing mentoring for executive and middle managers is one way to not only develop them, but also to demonstrate the behaviors for them to emulate.

Institutional mentoring systems and structures can take varied forms. The intention is to embed the value of mentoring into the organizational and unit behaviors. Again, this can be done at the organizational or at the local level. One example of a mentoring system and structure would be implementing an annual evaluation system that embeds "developing others" as an evaluation component. This is one concrete way to communicate to staff and leadership that their actions to develop other people are valued and are a performance metric. Another example would be a mentoring newsletter where stories from protégés are submitted about their nurse mentor and how their mentors helped them to achieve career goals. Units can create story boards where nurses can post when they "caught someone mentoring." Obviously, there are various ways that the value of mentoring can be embedded into the organizational and unit systems and structures. The key is that these systems and structures exist and that they stem from an organizational value of mentoring.

Formal mentoring programs are gaining in popularity. The advantage to a formal mentoring program is that it provides structure for mentoring to be enacted in the workplace. Leaders must evaluate the quality of any formal mentoring program before adopting it. Many formal mentoring programs that are in place today are essentially a series of meeting checklists with time frames for when meetings should happen. Many of these programs do not include the content and purpose for the mentoring meeting and the mentoring relationship. I call this type of program *mentoring by checklist*. Research shows that *mentoring by checklist* doesn't work, but rather achieving high quality mentoring relationships is really what matters (Jakubik, 2008, Jakubik et al, 2011). It is essential that when leaders adopt formal mentoring programs they assure that they are designed to provide the values-based benefits of mentoring that the organization seeks to achieve.

Informal mentoring is a powerful organizational phenomenon. Research demonstrates that the majority of nurses who are mentored will go on to become mentors (Jakubik, 2008, Jakubik et al, 2011, Jakubik et al, 2013). So the act of mentoring is two-fold: to develop the individual protégé and to build future mentors through mentoring. Informal mentoring can also be promoted by leaders who role model mentoring. Leaders who successfully embed the value of mentoring in their workforces, promote informal mentoring through the systems and structures they build around mentoring.

Career Development Exercise

1. List the mentoring systems, structures, and/or programs that your organization has in place:

_____

_____

_____

2. How would you rate the level at which the organization/organizational leaders value mentoring (e.g. high, moderate, low)?

_____

_____

_____

3. What could you as an organizational leader do to facilitate mentoring from an organizational perspective?

_____

_____

_____

Chapter 5
Membership and Leadership: Nursing Specialty Professional Organizations

Part 1: Nurses

Nursing specialty professional organizations can be a powerful force in the development of a nurse's career. They provide a forum for specialty nurses from across the globe to share knowledge, disseminate research, address problems facing the nursing specialty and its patient population, and create a professional network within the nursing specialty.

Nursing specialty professional organizations offer concrete benefits to members such as newsletter and journal subscriptions, conference discounts, professional development opportunities and networking opportunities. However, these stated, concrete benefits are only the beginning. Career benefits increase with increasing involvement in a nursing specialty professional organization. Let's take a more in-depth look at all of the benefits for joining and getting involved in your nursing specialty professional organization.

Informing Nursing Practice

Your nursing specialty professional organization's annual conference is the forum where the latest evidence about your specialty is disseminated through national and international experts on topics specific to the specialty. It is truly a place to get the most up to date information to inform practice as many experts disseminate research through poster and oral presentations before the information is available in print in peer-refereed journals or text books. These conferences provide an opportunity for you to compare your own practice to others as practices are shared through poster and oral presentations.

A subscription to the organization's peer-refereed journal is typically a benefit of membership. This journal may be provided either in print or in electronic format or both. This journal is a major resource for you to inform your practice throughout the year about the latest evidence in your nursing specialty. In addition to research articles, the journal may also present columns on hot topics, case studies, and practice and/or education projects or creative solutions to clinical problems.

Committee and Leadership Opportunities

Nursing specialty professional organizations are always looking for opportunities to cultivate new leadership. Typically, there is a movement up the ranks in organizational leadership from leadership in a local chapter, to membership in a national committee, to chairing a national committee, to being elected to the board of directors.

Local chapters of your nursing specialty professional organization provide an avenue to get nurses in your region involved with the work of the organization. These local chapters frequently are challenged with turn-over of chapter leadership and the need to recruit new members and new leaders to serve on the board of directors. Your local chapter is an excellent place to get involved in your nursing specialty professional organization. It is a way to really make a difference in spreading the mission of the organization to nurses in your local area.

Another way to grow as a leader in your nursing specialty professional organization is to join a national committee. There are typically committees in areas such as education, research, public policy, and chapter development. These committees generally meet via conference call throughout the year and then host a live meeting at the annual conference. And these committees often have directives from the board of directors for projects to address throughout the year. Typically, the committee chair works to inform the board of directors about the work of the committee through meeting minutes and an annual report at the annual conference where members are also invited.

The board of directors is generally filled with those members who have become involved in and led the nursing specialty professional organization through local chapter and/or national committee participation. The organization will hold elections for positions on the board of directors regularly (e.g. every 2 years) in accordance with the by-laws. Members of the board of directors typically come from across the globe and represent a range of academic preparation (BSN, MSN, PhD, etc.) and roles in nursing (staff nurse, clinical nurse specialist, nurse educator, nurse administrator). So if joining the leadership of your nursing specialty professional organization is a goal, start by joining and getting involved at the committee level.

Choosing a Professional Organization

The first nursing specialty professional organization to join in your nursing career is the one that is most closely aligned to your nursing clinical practice (e.g. medical-surgical nursing, pediatric nursing, etc.) However, once you grow and subspecialize in your career, you may also want to join a more role-focused organization. For instance, nurse managers should join the American Organization for Nurse Executives (AONE).

Career Development Exercise

1. List the personal benefits for you to belong to a nursing specialty professional organization:

_____

_____

2. List the nursing specialty professional organizations of which you are a member:

_____

_____

3. List the nursing specialty professional organization of which you are <u>not</u> a member, but would be beneficial for you to join:

_____

_____

4. Are you an active member of your local or national nursing specialty professional organization(s) by volunteering for committee leadership, or other volunteer activity? If so, list your activities. If not, list at least 2 ways you could get more involved.

_____

_____

_____

Part II: Hospitals

Membership and leadership in nursing specialty professional organizations not only provides career enhancement for individual nurses but also provides prestige and fulfillment of organizational goals including credentialing and portfolio development for the organization. Additionally, nurses who become leaders in their nursing specialty professional organizations showcase their hospital and provide both outreach and marketing on behalf of the hospital. It is, therefore, critical that hospitals do their part to support individual nurses in becoming involved in these professional organizations. It is truly a win-win for the nurse and the hospital.

Role Modeling

Membership and leadership in nursing specialty professional organizations is a professional activity that must be role modeled by hospital nursing leadership. When novice and advanced beginner nurses see that the hospital nursing leaders are active, contributing members of their nursing specialty professional organization, that sets the stage for an organizational culture that values membership and leadership in nursing specialty professional organizations. Leaders in nursing are really called to give back to the profession through their involvement and leadership at the local and national levels of their nursing specialty professional organizations. So the first step for hospitals in supporting career development though nursing specialty professional organizations is to assess the degree of current participation in these organizations among the hospital's nursing leadership at all levels (middle management, executive administration, education, and advanced practice.)

Providing Resources

Hosting Onsite Meetings

Nursing specialty professional organization local chapters need locations to host their board meetings, membership meetings, and CE events. These meetings are typically fairly small, are hosted in the evening after business hours, or on a Saturday. These are times when hospital conference rooms are typically available. Hosting the membership meeting and CE event onsite at your hospital may encourage nurses working at your facility to attend and also sets a tone that your hospital supports the important work of these nursing specialty professional organizations.

Providing Faculty

Providing faculty to present CE content at the local chapter meetings is another way to not only support the work of the local chapter but also to showcase your hospital's talent. The local chapter is in constant need of speakers for CE to provide new and up-to-date content for its members, so this is an ideal way to support the local chapter, encourage your nursing leadership to present, and show your hospital's organizational commitment to maintaining an active role in the work of the local chapter.

Providing Board Membership/Leadership

One of the most challenging tasks at both the local and national levels is to bring in a constant stream of nursing leaders to fill board of director positions to lead the organization. Hospitals that have adopted an organizational culture which supports nursing specialty professional organizations should support their nursing leadership in serving in these roles on boards of directors. There are clear benefits to the individual nurse leader who serves in terms of leadership development and networking. But there are also benefits to the hospital of demonstrating contribution to the nursing profession, showcasing the hospital's leadership talent, and overall marketing.

Financial Support

Organizational values are reflected in their bottom line. Organizations typically financially support what they value. Membership in a professional organization requires an annual dues payment which can vary widely. Hospitals should consider allocating tuition reimbursement funds for the reimbursement of membership dues for nursing specialty professional organizations. Furthermore, hospital nursing leadership should partner with nursing specialty professional organizations to create "membership dues packages" that allow an organization to enroll some or all of its nurses as members for a significant discount. There is power in large numbers.

Reward and Recognition

Membership in a nursing specialty professional organization should be considered as a reward and recognition incentive. Rather than umbrellas, beach towels, coffee mugs or other gifts during *Nurses' Week*, why not consider a 3-month trial membership to a nursing specialty professional organization? The nursing specialty professional organizations want access to nurses in hospitals and hospitals what their nurses to be members, so this partnership is truly a *win-win*. It will just take some creativity on both parts.

Hospitals should take opportunities to display and to recognize those nurses in the hospital who are leading in nursing specialty professional organizations. Recognition might include a story in a hospital paper or electronic newsletter. *Nursing Grand Rounds* should showcase activities in nursing specialty professional organizations on an annual basis. This can be a panel of those who lead at the local and national level talking about their nursing specialty professional organization and their particular activities in them. *Nurses' Week* is an ideal time to sponsor this type of *Nursing Grand Rounds* presentation.

Career Development Exercise

1. Does your hospital possess leaders who are active in nursing specialty professional organizations?

_____

2. What is the rate of membership among nursing staff in nursing specialty professional organizations (e.g. high, moderate, low)?

_____

3. How does your hospital structurally (e.g. policies, procedures, systems) support nurses in becoming members in nursing specialty professional organizations?

_____

_____

_____

4. How can you as an organizational leader support nurses to join and participate in nursing professional organizations?

_____

_____

_____

_____

Chapter 6
Building a Professional Network

Part I: Nurses

Networking is a powerful *career development tool* that can open many doors for a nurse both within his or her hospital as well as in the larger nursing profession.

Networking Within the Organization

One of the best ways to start to build your professional network within your hospital is to join a committee through your unit's shared governance structure. Shared governance is an administrative model that provides for staff nurse input into decision making at the unit and at the hospital level. Choose the committee (education, practice, operations, research, etc.) whose work is aligned with your interests. Getting involved in a committee will expose you to nurses on your unit who work different shifts than you do and will allow you to share ideas and receive information about the work of your unit and the hospital. These unit based committees typically appoint or elect a chairperson who represents the unit in the larger hospital-based committee meeting which generally meets monthly. This is an opportunity to develop leadership skills and to further network with other nurses on the hospital-based committee.

Networking Outside of the Organization

Nursing Specialty Professional Organizations

Joining a nursing specialty professional organization can be a tremendous opportunity to build a professional network. Through your involvement in your nursing specialty professional organization, you have the opportunity to build your world in nursing beyond the walls of your workplace. You can do this through attendance at the annual convention, participation in your local chapter, participation in the national organization's committees, and joining the national list serve.

Annual Conference Attendance

Attending your nursing specialty professional organization's annual convention provides a great opportunity to meet nurses from across the country. When you attend the national convention make sure to bring business cards with your name, credentials, title, employer, and email address. When others give you their business card, take a moment to write down on the back of their card something about them in order to jog your memory later on when you have a pile of business cards.

If you attend a presentation on a topic that is particularly important to your clinical practice and would like to follow up with the speaker and/or add the speaker to your professional contacts, introduce yourself to the speaker after the presentation and ask for his or her business card. Speakers often list their email address on their first or last power point slide.

Many of the national experts who are authors of the nursing specialty text books and editors of the specialty's peer-refereed journals are leaders in the nursing specialty professional organization and are present for you to meet. Additionally, these authors and editors will often mentor attendees and provide support for career development and professional goal achievement such as getting published. It is often exhilarating to meet in-person the authors of the text books you have on the shelf back in your workplace. These authors are often available to talk with you and to share their expertise with you at the annual conference.

Local Chapter Participation

Joining and becoming involved in your nursing specialty professional organization's local chapter can be a great way to expand your nursing world while building your leadership skills and your contribution to the national organization, all at the local level. One of the best parts about membership of the local chapter is that you will have the opportunity to meet other nurses from units in your own hospital and from other hospitals in the region.

I have personally experienced the power of a local chapter in transforming the relationships among hospitals in a region through breaking down existing silos and promoting team work. My own experience serving as a leader at the local chapter level was that nurses working at competing hospitals became colleagues and eventually friends. Ultimately, this group of nurses led a regional conference that brought nurses from across the region together to learn, share, and network annually. This group of leaders at the local chapter level literally transformed a region through their ability to network and break down silos through that professional network. As of this writing, this regional conference is in its 11th year with over 400 nurses attending annually.

National Committee Participation

Committee participation at the national level provides an opportunity to meet nurses from across the country that are interested in serving particular interests of the board of directors through a committee's work. These committees typically meet in-person at the annual conference and then meet regularly throughout the year via conference call. Because of the regular meeting schedule, members of the committee really do get to know each other and build a professional network through the work of the committee. Additionally, a member of the board of directors is often a liaison to the committee, so this is also an opportunity to get to know a board member and to showcase your talents to that board member.

One of the great advantages to networking through your professional organization, whether it's through the live conference, local chapter, or committee participation, is that you have the opportunity to create a professional identity that is separate from your job or role and the politics that go with that back in your hospital. This can be a huge advantage in building a network that extends beyond the roles and political strata of your hospital.

National List Serve Subscription

The national list serve of your nursing specialty professional organization can be a tremendous resource for gaining information from your nursing colleagues from across the country and even the world. This list serve is a place where nurses can post questions about clinical, education, or other topics. Frequently nurses will post questions about experiences with a particular product or service. It is sort of like asking your colleague on the unit for his or her opinion or experience, except that you post the question to hundreds or even thousands of nurses within your specialty with one email to the list serve. This can be a very valuable tool to support your clinical practice. A word to the wise: If you join a list serve, it is a good idea to do so on an email account that is not your routine email since questions and answers occur daily which has a tendency to flood one's email in-box. Some list serves are more technologically sophisticated than others, but this is a common problem of which to be aware.

Career Development Exercise

1. List the personal benefits for you to building your professional network:

_____

_____

_____

_____

2. List the ways in which you are currently building your professional network:

_____

_____

_____

_____

3. List at least 2 additional ways that you could further build your professional network:

_____

_____

_____

_____

Part II: Hospitals

Hospitals have an important role in supporting their nurses to expand their professional network. Nursing leaders within hospitals from middle managers to senior executives should consider building systems and structures that support nurses in networking within their hospital, the region, and the larger nursing subspecialty at the national level.

Networking Within the Organization

Shared governance structures can support nurses to build a professional network within their hospital. The purpose of shared governance is to provide an administrative model where nurses can have input into decision-making. Committees within the shared governance models typically reflect the work of the unit and the department as in: education, practice, research/evidence-based practice, and operations/management. Shared governance committees are excellent forums for nurses to participate in the work of their hospital and also to meet colleagues from other areas of the hospital. These colleagues often become friends and mentors.

Hospitals that require each nurse to join a unit-based shared governance committee provide a basis for their nurses to get involved and to network within and beyond their own unit or area of employment. Shared governance committees, therefore, provide a really excellent way for nurses to network within their unit/area and within the larger organization.

Networking Outside of the Organization

Hospitals ideally want to attract and develop nursing talent who can go beyond the hospital walls and act as excellent representatives on behalf of the organization. Networking outside of the organization has several advantages for hospitals:

✓ recruiting top talent to join the organization

✓ building the organization's reputation by sharing best practices

- ✓ benchmarking best practices, equipment, etc. used in other organizations
- ✓ expanding the organization's overall reach and influence

Career Development Exercise

1. What degree of value (high, moderate, low) do you believe that internal networking within the hospital has for nurses and for the broader organization?

_____

2. How does your hospital structurally (e.g. policies, systems, structures) promote networking <u>within</u> the organization?

_____

_____

3. How does your hospital structurally (e.g. policies, systems, structures) promote networking <u>outside</u> of the organization?

_____

_____

4. List at least 2 ways that you as an organizational leader could work to promote networking among nurses <u>within</u> and <u>outside</u> of your organization:

_____

_____

_____

_____

Chapter 7
Presenting Your Work

Part I: Nurses

Developing skills as a presenter is a significant component of career development for a nurse. Benefits of presenting include: giving back to the profession, intrinsic reward, promotion opportunities, and external recognition.

Presentation is an important component of disseminating nursing knowledge and to helping others in nursing to benefit from your expertise. The most important first step in developing skills for presentation is to hone your specialty knowledge. As a presenter, you will be seen as an expert in the topic or project you are presenting, so becoming knowledgeable in your area is a key ingredient to becoming a presenter. The next important step is to study and seek mentoring in the art and skill of presenting in various formats (poster or oral).

Opportunities for poster and oral presentations are available at hospital poster sessions, local conferences, and national conferences. These opportunities are generally available either by invitation or blinded abstract submission. Presentations should be viewed as on a continuum from novice to expert beginning with poster presentations at the hospital or local level and advancing to oral presentations at national conferences.

Poster Presentations

Poster presentations provide an opportunity to share information about a clinical, education, or research project. The format provides a unique opportunity to share and discuss projects with conference participants as they view your poster. Poster presentations are often a stepping stone to the development of an oral presentation or manuscript for publication in a scholarly journal.

Poster presentation skills can best be honed by starting with a poster presentation at a hospital-based or local conference and then advancing to a poster presentation at a national conference. Poster presentations can be created simply and inexpensively and they can also be very sophisticated and rather expensive to have printed by a professional printer. A simple and inexpensive way to create a poster presentation is to use PowerPoint slides that are printed and posted on a poster board or easel. Of course, a printer can design and/or print your poster for you. There are numerous print-based and web-based resources to support poster presenters in developing a poster for presentation as well as for presenting it. My favorite resource for posters printing and related equipment such as poster carrying cases is the website www.posters4research.com. My experience is that they provide high-quality, affordable products and printing services.

Oral Presentations

Oral presentations provide a unique opportunity to share knowledge with an audience in an in-depth way due to the time allotted for an oral presentation. Oral presentations require refinement of oral communication and audiovisual skills and, therefore, provide an excellent opportunity to develop skills in public speaking. This presentation format affords nurses the opportunity to share knowledge, lead discussion, and answer questions about a particular area of expertise. Oral presentations are an additional stepping stone to the development of manuscripts for publication in a scholarly journal.

Career Development Exercise

1. List the personal benefits for you to present your work either as a poster or oral presentation:

_____

_____

2. List the benefits to your organization for you to present your work either as a poster or oral presentation:

_____

_____

3. List at least 1 project (education, clinical, research) that you are/were involved in that could be the topic of a presentation:

_____

_____

4. List at least 3 steps you could take to pursue a presentation (poster or oral) about your project:

_____

_____

_____

_____

Part II: Hospitals

Supporting nurses to present in a variety of forums and formats is a valuable way for hospitals to develop nursing talent as well as to enhance the organization's annual reporting of nursing scholarly activities. It is important that hospitals put in place systems and structures to support nurses to present poster and oral presentations within the hospital, regionally, and nationally.

An Opportunity and a Responsibility

Presenting an oral or poster presentation at a regional or national conference is a huge opportunity and also a huge responsibility. Hospitals owe it to their nurses to support them in this experience and nurses owe it to their hospitals to be prepared to be the best ambassador of the organization they can possibly be. This partnership requires both participants to do their part. Organizations must be clear in what they are able to provide in terms of support as well as what the expectations are in terms of the nurse's role. And the nurse must gain an understanding of what is involved and expected in representing the hospital in this way at a regional or national conference.

Nursing leaders should consider the level of support that the nursing department gives to nurses who present. There are several issues to consider when making the decision about allocating resources for poster and oral presentations. Questions to consider are:

What is the degree of value placed on poster and oral presentation by the hospital?

Organizations that are learning-oriented will place emphasis on the need for nurses to present and share their knowledge and best practices. Some hospitals place a hierarchy on the type of presentation. For instance poster presentations may be geared toward national conferences and oral presentations for regional conferences.

What is the expectation of the presenter?

Hospitals will have most success if they are clear with nurses about what the expectation and value is regarding poster and oral presentation. Nursing department leaders can do simple things like encouraging nurses to submit abstracts for particular conferences where the hospital would like to be represented and where there are resources to support the presenter. Nursing department leaders should mentor nurses who will be presenting regionally or nationally to understand what it means to represent the hospital including appropriate business dress and how to conduct oneself when representing the hospital at a conference. This may seem like a simple thing, however, a nurse who has never presented a poster or attended a regional or national conference might not be aware of the expectations regarding professional dress and that they will be asked to stand by their poster and answer questions of conference participants and poster judges. It is important that this expectation is clear so that the nurse is supported in being successful and also so that the hospital is well-positioned by the nurse who is representing the organization.

Systems and Structures

Systems and structures should be put in place to support the nurse who will be presenting either a poster or oral presentation. But these do not need to be complicated or expensive.

Human Resources

Educational Support/Mentorship

It is helpful to partner the nurse presenter with a nurse educator or seasoned poster presenter to provide support and mentoring. This is particularly important for novice nurse presenter who might not know where to begin the process of putting a presentation together. This also creates a professional development opportunity for the mentor in this relationship to grow in his or her own role as teacher and coach. The mentor should provide an overview of what is involved in the creation of the presentation and provide some helpful resources for the presenter to use.

Physical/Financial Resources

Time

It is essential that the nurse and the hospital achieve clarity from the start about how time will be allocated for the creation of the presentation. An issue to consider is whether the presentation be created entirely outside of work, entirely during paid work time, or some combination of the two. These are important factors for the organization and the nurse to consider. To some extent, as nurses develop in their roles and take on more presentation opportunities, the time does spill over into personal, unpaid time. However, this is a fact that novice presenters might not recognize and should not be taken for granted by the nurse presenter or by nursing department leadership. Ideally, a balance of paid time and personal time dedicated to preparing for the presentation is the right balance to strike.

Poster Development and Printing

Poster presentations can range from print outs of power point slides that are mounted directly on the poster easel provided by the conference to glossy 8 X 4 foot posters costing as much as $300 and literally everything in between. It is important to discuss with the presenter what the physical resources and financial resources are for creating the presentation. Physical resources would include access to a computer to create PowerPoint slides or to actually create the poster within it; access to a printer only to print the print-ready file; or even a full service graphic art department that can create the entire poster file and print it. Obviously the particular physical resource selected for the project affects the budget dollars required. These are important discussions to have up front, in the beginning so that the expectations are clear for the individual nurse and the organization.

Conference Support

Since budgets are not infinite, hospital leadership must consider what resources can reasonably be allocated to supporting a nurse's attendance at a regional or national conference. Equally important, is that the organization develop a guideline for how such financial support will be allocated. As an example, many hospitals will provide more financial support for conference attendance for nurses who are presenting an oral rather than a poster presentation because an oral presentation is considered more prestigious and, therefore, more valuable to the organization's resume. And while there is a hierarchy in terms of presentations (e.g. poster, oral concurrent abstract submission, oral keynote by invitation), an organization that aims to build its repertoire of presentations and presenters might encourage and support poster presenters due to their capacity to develop novice presenters and to become oral presentations and publications in the future.

Alternatively, priority may be placed on allocating budget dollars to support a presenter at a national versus a regional convention regardless of the presentation format due to the fact that national conference presentations are generally considered more prestigious. On the other hand, an organization might decide that presenting multiple poster presentations at a regional conference is a low-cost way to increase the number of presentations giving more nurses an opportunity to present while getting the biggest bang for the buck.

Recognition

Recognition can be one of the most valuable and often zero cost ways of supporting a nurse presenter. Being recognized by organizational leaders in either formal or informal ways can be a huge satisfier for the individual nurse presenter and often creates excitement among fellow nursing colleagues, all while setting an example for the value the organization holds on nurses presenting their work. Recognition can take various formats. The remainder of this chapter presents a few examples.

A Dry Run

One of my favorite ways to recognize a nurse who is going to a conference to present is to host a breakfast or lunch in a conference room where the nurse can actually conduct the presentation for his or her colleagues while they listen and have a bite to eat. This accomplishes several things. First, it is an opportunity for the nurse to actually practice a dry run of the presentation in a familiar and supportive environment. Second, it creates an opportunity for members of the organization to learn about the nurse's work and that he or she is going to be presenting it at a conference. This is important because in our busy work lives, often times we don't know the good work that our colleagues are engaged in and presenting at outside conferences. Third, providing a forum for the nurse presenter to practice the presentation in front of a live audience is generally a big confidence boost. It allows the nurse to work out any kinks in the presentation and to feel more comfortable on the regional or national stage.

Recognition in a Public Forum

You have probably heard the age old management saying: *Recognize in public, reprimand in private.* It is amazing how much a public recognition at a meeting or other forum can mean. Nurse leaders can start a behavior where certain meetings or public forums start with a reading of the list of professional activities that nurses engaged in since the last meeting. These announcements could be made at staff meetings, council meetings, or even *Nursing Grand Rounds.*

Flyer or Website Posting

A paper or electronic flyer announcing the nurse's upcoming presentation is an excellent way to recognize this achievement. If your organization's infrastructure allows, you might add a nursing accomplishments page to the website where nurses' professional activities are listed.

Department Annual Report

The nursing department's annual report is definitely a place that organizational leaders should assure that nurses' professional activities are listed. This is a way for the organization to highlight their human resource talent and to quantify the level of professional nursing activities that are being accomplished.

Career Development Exercise

1. What degree of value (high, moderate, low) does presenting professional work have for you personally and for the hospital?

_____

2. How does your hospital structurally (e.g. resources, policies, systems, structures) promote presentations at onsite or local/regional conferences?

_____

_____

3. How does your hospital structurally (e.g. resources, policies, systems, structures) promote presentations at national conferences?

_____

_____

4. List at least 2 ways that you as an organizational leader could work to increase the level of support for individual nurses to present their work:

_____

_____

Chapter 8
Getting Published

Part I: Nurses

Getting published can seem like a daunting task. And it can be. However, if it is a professional goal for you there are some concrete ways that you can start. It is typically best to find a mentor and to start with a smaller publication project first. For instance, you might first publish in a newsletter before working gradually toward the big goal of primary authorship in a scholarly journal. Each of your publications, no matter how small, is a stepping stone towards the next publication.

Publication Formats

Newsletters

Nursing newsletters are available at the unit and hospital level. Additionally, the local chapter and national specialty professional organization generally have newsletters. These are avenues for getting started in your role as an author. These are media forums that are typically looking for submissions and provide you with the assistance of a newsletter editor to refine your submission. And frequently the word count requirements for a newsletter submission are small in the range of 1-4 paragraphs. So it is a manageable project to begin your work as an author.

Scholarly Journal Article Co-Authorship

An excellent way to hone your writing skills is to join a writing group under the tutelage of a seasoned primary author. There are frequently nurse researchers and clinicians in hospitals who are looking for team members to assist with the projects and to be part of the writing team. I've done this several times as a primary author and I can tell you that it is terrific to have the assistance of other nurses to get the writing done. And my protégés in writing have told me that it was a great way to learn the writing and publication process.

One way to get started with finding a writing team is to alert your hospital's nursing education, practice, and/or research department that you are looking to get started in getting published and would like to be part of a writing team. Another option is to let those clinical experts that you work with know that you are looking for a writing partner to learn from and assist in the writing process.

Scholarly Journal Columns

Most scholarly journals have columns on particular topics of interest. These columns are not blindly peer-reviewed but rather are reviewed, accepted, and edited by the column's editor. This presents a unique opportunity. Column editors have ongoing needs for submissions for their column, so they are generally hungry for content. Additionally, because of the unique nature of the review and editing for column submissions, it sometimes easier to get published in a column and affords you the one on one mentorship and expertise of the column editor.

Primary Author Journal Articles

Primary authorship of an article in a peer-refereed journal is really the pinnacle of authorship. Typically, the timeline from the start of writing to publication in the scholarly journal can take about two years (with wide variability). You can see why I recommend that you work up to this publication format.

Getting Started

Your first step is to decide what to write about. This requires that you examine what you have expertise in and what the holes are in the literature. So make a list of topics you could write about and then perform an electronic literature search to see if there is a need in the literature for your topic.

Once you have a topic, you need to create an outline and working title for your manuscript. (Your written work is called a manuscript while you are writing and submitting it and an article after it is published.) At the same time, it is a good idea to identify the journal to which you wish to submit your manuscript. To determine which journal is best, consider whom you are aiming to reach. Are you targeting the clinical nurse at the bedside; the educator; the nurse manger; the nurse researcher? Knowing your audience should assist you to narrow down your list of potential journals to consider. Next take a look at the types of articles that appear in each of the journals on your short list and consider which type of article best represents the writing style and format for the manuscript you wish to write.

Once you've identified your topic, working title, and journal for submission, you should write a query letter to the journal's editor to determine whether the editor has interest in a manuscript on your topic. (Typically, this letter is submitted via email.) This is not required, but I do think it is an important step. You'd be surprised at the responses you may get. At times, you will have an editor who is very eager to receive your manuscript and at other times you will receive a response from an editor who is not interested and thinks your topic is either uninteresting or unoriginal. If you get a response from an editor who is not interested in your manuscript topic, you can either ask how you could refine the topic to meet the journal's needs or find another journal who has interest in your topic.

Writing

You've identified a manuscript topic and a journal with interest in your manuscript. Now it is time to write. Before you start, make sure that you consult the author guidelines for the journal you have selected for submission in order to understand their guidelines about formatting and manuscript length. Make sure you follow these guidelines to the letter. If you don't, you will put the acceptance of your manuscript at risk. Some journal editors and reviewers will automatically reject manuscripts that don't conform to the journal's guidelines.

If you are writing in a group, it is a good idea to set up twice monthly meetings to divide up the work and provide periodic updates on work status. As the primary author, you should ask team members to submit their work to you. You should copy and paste their submissions in to the body of the manuscript, save under the article name and current date, and send the updated manuscript out to the team members several days before each meeting. (You want team members to have time to read the updated manuscript.) If you are writing as a solo author, it is a good idea to create a timeline with work product goals and to carve out weekly or daily time to write.

Whether or not you are writing in a team or solo, you will need to carve out time to write in order to achieve your writing deadlines. Many novice authors make the mistake of saying they will write when they can "find time." This is a trap. You don't "find time" to write. Writing literally needs to be carved into your day or your week. Make it a priority and schedule it.

Personally, I always have at least one, and often two writing projects going at any point in time. And I find that the best way to get writing projects done is to schedule it into my week. I like to write in the morning before anyone in my home is awake and before my work day has officially started. I make a pot of coffee, sit in my favorite chair under a blanket, and get to writing. My goal is typically to write for 1-2 hours, 1-2 times per week. Some weeks I accomplish more and some weeks less, but I have a goal and it keeps me on track. I actually have a "to do list" on my table next to my favorite writing chair and always have the writing goals list for the week written there to keep me motivated and on track.

Reviewing

Once you have written your very best draft of your manuscript, I suggest you step away from it for a few days or even 1-2 weeks to get some space from it. This space will give you a renewed perspective for your final review of it. Then review the manuscript a final time and make any necessary edits.

Once you have your personal best version of the manuscript, there is one more step before submission to the journal. That final step is to conduct an internal review using your own experts. To do this, you need to reach out to 1-3 trusted people in your personal and professional life to ask them to review and give you feedback. Give each of them 10 days to get back to you so there is a clear deadline for receiving feedback. It is a good idea to have 2 professionals who are good writers but have different perspectives. So for instance have a nurse researcher or educator review your manuscript and also a nurse clinician. I also like to find an editor who is a non-nurse. I have a few family members who are top notch writers and not nurses, so I almost always have one of them edit my manuscript as well. You'd be surprised at the different, yet high quality feedback these varied perspectives and talents can provide. Many experienced authors use this process of internal review to achieve the absolute best manuscript for submission to the journal.

Once you have all of these internal reviewers' feedback, you should make your final edits. You will be amazed at how much better your manuscript is now that it has your very best work as well as the input of two to three of your personal and professional colleagues. Now it is time to submit to the journal and wait. Refer to the journal's website for typical response time post-manuscript submission. Typically, the waiting time takes about 3 months with wide variability.

When you receive feedback from the journal editor, it will be one of the following responses:
- ✓ accept without revision
- ✓ accept with revision
- ✓ revise and resubmit
- ✓ reject

Acceptance with or without revisions is certainly the easiest and most encouraging response. Simply make any changes and respond to the editor with the revised manuscript and a cover letter explaining how you've responded to the request for revisions. If you receive a "revise and resubmit" response, do not be discouraged. This response means that the journal is interested in your manuscript but it needs significant changes before being re-reviewed. Many writers are discouraged by this response and don't revise and resubmit.

This is a mistake. Even if the manuscript was rejected by the journal editor that does not mean that the manuscript will not eventually get published. Pay attention to the reason why the manuscript was rejected. If it simply was not a good fit for that journal, perhaps a different journal would be interested in the manuscript. If the issue was related to poor writing quality, perhaps a writing coach would be a good resource to assist you in revising the manuscript.

Career Development Exercise

1. List the personal benefits for you to become a published author:

_____

_____

_____

_____

2. List the benefits to your hospital for you to become a published author:

_____

_____

_____

_____

3. List at least 1 topic that you could write about:

_____

_____

_____

_____

4. List at least 3 steps you could take to pursue writing about your selected topic:

_____

_____

_____

_____

Part 2: Hospitals

Supporting nurses to get published has value to any organization. It raises the academic prestige of the nursing department when there are published authors. It also is a prestigious accomplishment that reflects on the quality of the nurses in the organization but also the overall quality of the organization itself. Hospitals can put in place systems and structures that support nurses to get started in the publication process.

Systems and Structures

If publishing is a goal for the nursing department, then it is important that educational systems and structures are set up to promote the attainment of this individual and organizational goal. Few people become published alone without support and direction. Let's examine a few examples of ways in which the organization can support the publication process.

Education/Mentoring for Publication

Informal Forums

Nurses who are considering getting started with writing and publication need concrete information about the publishing process. This can take many formats. One option would be to pair a novice nurse author with a seasoned author for meeting and direction. This would provide for long-term support and direction in the publishing process.

There are private writing coaches who can be hired (for a fee) to guide you through the publication process. Typically, this option makes the most sense for a nurse who does not have access to any resources within the hospital for publication.

Formal Classes

Another option would be to provide a *Getting Published* class taking place bi-weekly over an extended period of time (e.g. several months) where a seasoned author could teach novices how to move from topic idea, to journal selection, to query letter, to drafts writing, to internal review, to completed manuscript for submission. This format would, of course, require that the organization has access to a seasoned author, either internally or externally, who could teach this class. Some national conferences provide pre-conference workshops on *Getting Published*.

Writing Teams

One of my favorite ways to write a scholarly article in nursing is in a writing team. Typically, this format involves one or more experienced nurse authors who wish to partner with novice and/or advanced beginner writers with the goal of gaining their time and assistance with research, literature review, writing sections of the article in exchange for mentoring in the process of writing and publishing. These writing teams can be so productive because the work is divided amongst a half-dozen people.

When putting together a writing team, it's generally best not to make them much bigger than around 6 people. And sometimes members of the team are simply there to learn and not to be authors on the publication. For instance student nurses might conduct the literature search and some articles for the literature review section of the manuscript and thus would be appropriately acknowledged on the publication but not co-authors on the publication. Writing teams work well when they are large enough to share the workload, but not so large that it becomes difficult to manage.

One of the most important things to establish in the writing group is the division of work and the order of authorship. The experienced nurse author should assure that only those who actually contributed to the work and the writing are named as authors. The conversation around the division of workload and authorship is an important discussion to have at the outset. Additionally, these writing groups are typically teaching-learning forums so it's important to take time while meeting to explain the writing and publication process.

Career Development Exercise

1. What degree of value (high, moderate, low) does publishing professional work have for you personally and for your hospital?

_____

2. What percentage of nurses in your hospital are published (high, moderate, low)?

_____

3. How does your hospital structurally (e.g. resources, policies, systems, structures) promote nurses writing and becoming published?

_____

_____

_____

4. List at least 2 ways that you as an organizational leader could work to increase the level of organizational support for individual nurses to write and publish their work:

_____

_____

Chapter 9
Alphabet Soup:
Credentialing

Part 1: Nurses

Credentials sometimes feel like alphabet soup. However, it is important to signify the credentials you have earned as a professional nurse by listing your credentials after your name.

Credentials to Include

Minimally you must list on formal documents (chart notes, professional letters, etc.) any credentials required by the state board of nursing, such as minimum licensure for practice and any required certification for practice. It is also advisable to list any certifications or honorary degrees that were voluntary rather than required for practice. If these were important enough to earn in the first place, then they are important enough to list with your other credentials. A list of your academic degrees would typically be listed in the signature line of a letter but not in a chart note.

Ordering of Credentials

There is not an absolute right or wrong way to list one's nursing credentials. However, there are general guidelines to guide the process. *List credentials according to their degree of permanence from highest to lowest.* Following these guidelines one would order credentials in the following manner: academic degree, license, certifications. An *academic degree* is a permanent academic credential that cannot be lost once achieved. A *license* is granted by the state to allow for practice within a certain scope and can only be taken away by failure to renew it or through gross workplace misconduct. *Certification* within a nursing specialty area is granted after passing a certification exam and is valid for a period of years, requiring ongoing maintenance through continuing education and renewal through documentation of such and payment of a fee. Following these rules, Suzy Smith who has a bachelor's in nursing, licensure as a registered nurse, and is certified as an emergency nurse would document her professional credentials as Suzy Smith, BSN, RN, CEN. Nurses should not list prerequisite academic or licensure credentials that are prerequisites to a more advanced degree or license currently held. For instance, a nurse who holds a bachelor's and master's degree in nursing would not list his/her bachelor's degree. So when Suzy Smith earns her master's degree she would list her name as Suzy Smith, MSN, RN, CEN. Similarly, a nurse who achieves license as a nurse practitioner, would not list her registered nurse license since it is a prerequisite. So for instance, if Suzy Smith received her license as a certified registered nurse practitioner, she would list her name as Suzy Smith, MSN, CRNP, CEN.

Career Development Exercise

1. List your professional credentials:

_____

2. Look at your credentials above. How do you list them? Will you list them differently after reading this chapter?

_____

_____

3. Examining your credentials above, are there others you'd like to add? If so, which ones?

_____

_____

4. List at least 2 steps you could take to pursue adding to your list of credentials:

_____

_____

_____

_____

Part 2: Hospitals

Hospitals have an opportunity to set the milieu to support and value credentialing in nursing. Nursing department leadership should role model credentialing by seeking out higher education, advanced licensure and certification. Furthermore, leadership should promote and encourage their nurses to continually develop themselves by expanding their credentials and then being sure to list them after their names so that they are recognized for their accomplishments.

Career Development Exercise

1. What degree of value (high, moderate, low) does advanced credentialing have for you personally and for your hospital?

_____

2. How well (high, moderate, low) do nursing department leaders model achieving advanced credentialing?

_____

3. List at least 2 ways that you as a leader could work to increase the level of organizational support for individual nurses to pursue advanced credentialing:

_____

_____

_____

_____

Chapter 10
Keeping Track of Your Success: Creating A Career Toolbox

Part 1: Nurses

Nurses beginning their careers in nursing as novice nurses should be given a *career toolbox* either from their schools of nursing or their first employer. This is a tracking system that nurses can use throughout their careers to keep track of their career successes. So if you don't already have a career toolbox to organize your career achievements, you need to add that to your 'to do' list. Now we'll take a look at the components of your *career toolbox*.

Components of a Career Toolbox

Your career toolbox can by either a physical hanging files box of folders or an electronic file of folders. Either way, it should include the following folders:

1) licensure
2) certification
3) contact hours
4) presentations

5) good works (which I sometimes call a "cudos file") of compliments via email/letter
6) publication/authorship
7) annual employee evaluations

Certainly you can add other categories as appropriate. These files should be sub-divided by year to keep organized. Contents should include physical or electronically scanned documentation of progress toward the development of that category. A copy of your R.N. license should be placed in your *license folder*. A letter confirming any certifications and/or certification certificates should be placed in your *certification folder*. It is a good idea to keep a copy of certification requirements in that folder as well, for a quick reference. Contact hour certificates from conferences should be placed in the *contact hours folder*. It is a good idea to place the brochure or program agenda in that folder as well. Copies of flyers, brochures, and abstracts of poster and oral presentations should be placed in the *presentations folder*. Evaluation data from presentations should also be placed in that folder. Your *good works folder* should contain copies of emails or letters that you received to compliment you on your work product or service delivery. Copies of your publications (newsletters, columns, articles) should be placed in the *publications/authorship folder*. And the *annual employee evaluation folder* should contain a copy of every annual evaluation that you receive. I am amazed at how many nurses do not ask for a copy of their annual evaluation. This is documentation of your year's job performance. This can be used as support for future awards and job applications.

Resume vs. Professional Portfolio

Resume

A *resume* is a document that summarizes a nurse's academic preparation, certifications, skills, achievements, and professional activities. It is typically used to apply for a job or a promotion. It is a good idea to get assistance from either an experienced resume writer or an online resource to prepare your *resume*. The basic categories for a *resume* are: education; professional experiences; licenses and certifications; professional associations and memberships; presentations and publications; and honors and awards.

Professional Portfolio

A *professional portfolio* is a means of demonstrating professional competence through evidence of skills and professional achievements. There are two types of professional portfolios: (1.) *growth and development portfolio* and (2.) *best work portfolio.* The *growth and development portfolio* is a complete warehouse of all of your professional accomplishments and is typically for your eyes only. It includes: diploma copies, transcripts, contact hour certificates, inservices attended, copies of annual evaluations, letters/emails of support/ recommendations, summaries of significant patient cases, copies of professional work, brochures and handouts from presentations and/or inservices, publications, authored policies and procedures, and authored patient education plans and other patient education projects.

The *best work* portfolio is a collection taken from the *growth and development portfolio* that is submitted as evidence to support your application for a job, reward, or promotion. For instance, when applying for a position as a nurse educator on your unit, you would want to submit a *best work portfolio* of some of the educational materials and presentations you have created.

Career Development Exercise

1. What benefit would having a career tool box be for you and your career?

_____

_____

2. Do you have a career tool box? _____ If not, by what date can you create one and organize your professional accomplishments in it? Pick a date. Write it below. Put it on your calendar.

_____

3. What categories (organized by file folders) will you put in your career tool box? Make a list below.

_____

_____

_____

_____

_____

_____

_____

_____

Part 2: Hospitals

Once an organization has adopted a corporate value set of promoting nurses' career development and has begun to put in place measures to do just that, the next vital step is to provide nurses with information about how to keep track of it all. In the ideal world, nursing leaders would welcome new graduate nurses to their organizations and to their careers in nursing by handing them a physical or electronic *career tool box* with files that are organized by category to help each nurse keep track of his or her career successes in nursing. Hospitals have a role in not only providing and supporting systems and structures for nurses to develop their careers, but also in helping them to understand how to organize their many career successes.

Career Development Exercise

1. What degree of value (high, moderate, low) does organizing and managing one's nursing career have for you personally and for your hospital?

_____

_____

2. How well (high, moderate, low) do organizational leaders model keeping track of their own career development?

_____

_____

3. List at least 2 ways that you as an organizational leader could work to increase the level of organizational support and direction that nurses receive in terms of keeping track of their own career development by using tools such as a career tool box:

_____

_____

_____

_____

Bring Dr. Louise Jakubik, Nursing Career Development Expert, to Your Hospital!

Key Note Presentation:

- ❖ From Start to Finish: How to Build and Develop Your Career in Nursing

½-Day or 1-Day Workshop:

- ❖ Nursing Career Development: Strategies for Nurses and Hospitals to Build Careers in Nursing

Consultation:

- ❖ Unit/Organizational Nursing Career Development Needs Assessment

- ❖ Unit/Organizational Nursing Career Development Curriculum, Systems, and Structures Design

For more information contact Louise:
Phone: 610-656-0892
Email: Louise@nursebuilders.net
Website: www.nursebuilders.net

References

Jakubik, L.D. (2012). Development and testing of the Jakubik Mentoring Benefits Questionnaire among pediatric nurses. *Journal of Nursing Measurement*, 20 (2), 113-122(10). doi.org/10.1891/1061-3749.20.2.113

Jakubik, L. D. (2008). Jump Starting Your Nursing Career: Toolbox for Success. *Pennsylvania Nurse*, 4-7.

Jakubik, L.D. (2008). Mentoring beyond the first year: Predictors of mentoring benefits for pediatric staff nurse protégés. *Journal of Pediatric Nursing*, 23(4), 269–281.

Jakubik, L.D. (2007). The relationships among quality, quantity, and type of mentoring and mentoring benefits for pediatric staff nurse protégés (Doctoral dissertation). Available from ProQuest Dissertations and Theses database. (UMI No. 1283974231)

Jakubik, L.D., Eliades, A., Gavriloff, C., & Weese, M. (2011). Nurse mentoring study demonstrates a magnetic work environment: Predictors of mentoring benefits among pediatric nurses. Journal of Pediatric Nursing, 26(2), 156–164.

Weese, M.M.., Jakubik, L.D., Eliades, A., & Huth, J. (in press). The relationship between mentoring practices and mentoring benefits among pediatric staff nurse protégés.

Vance, C., & Olson, R. K. (1998). *The mentor connection in nursing*. New York: Springer.

Zey, M.G. (1993). *The mentor connection*. New Brunswick: Transaction Publishers.

www.ingramcontent.com/pod-product-compliance
Lightning Source LLC
Chambersburg PA
CBHW051507170526
45166CB00001B/430